HELLO, I'M

YOUR NAME HERE

HELLO, I'M

Pregnant!

— A JOURNAL —

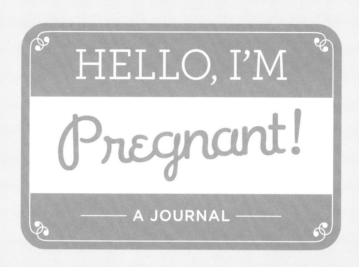

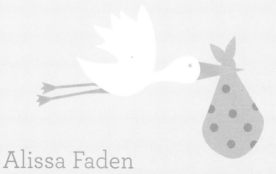

Alissa Faden

stewart, tabori & chang   new york

Hey, baby! Congratulations. You are going to be one hot mama! We've made this journal easy and fun to keep so that recording memories of your pregnancy will be a breeze.

Some days you'll have tons of energy and be inexplicably happy (that's the pregnant glow). For those days, there are pages with lots of space to be creative and a little crazy. Just let loose and jot down your thoughts about your bump and the changes you're going through physically and emotionally. Write about anything, from the love welling up inside you for your unborn child to your swelling breast size. It's up to you.

On days when you're feeling a little less energized, choose a page that has multiple choice or fill in the blank questions. Go in order or out of order within each trimester to suit your moods and your timeline. Just as every baby is not the same, not every pregnancy is the same. Use this book to match your needs. There's even an envelope in the back for you to tuck away small treasures like baby's hospital bracelet.

Just enjoy recording your bump-to-baby story—no need to labor over it. Labor comes later … And when the 9 months (well, actually a little longer) are over, you'll enjoy looking back through the special keepsake you've created.

Mommy
THAT'S ME

PASTE A PRE-PREGNANCY

PHOTO HERE

My full name is _____.

My nickname is _____.

I am _____ years old. (Shhh don't tell.)

I live in _____ with my _____.

This is my _____ pregnancy.

My other children (baby-to-be's brothers and sisters):

_____

_____

_____

_____

_____

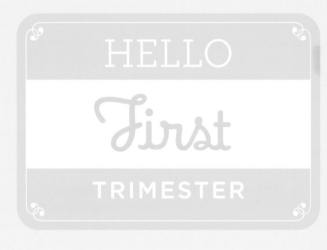

HELLO

First

TRIMESTER

PROOF positive

WHEN I FIRST SUSPECTED I WAS PREGNANT

Date: /   /   Time: Location:

Describe the circumstances:

_____

_____

_____

_____

_____

If you took a home pregnancy test, highlight the result here.   ➕ ➖

WHEN THE DOCTOR CONFIRMED IT

Date: /   /   Time: Location:

My reaction:

_____

_____

_____

Father-to-Be's reaction: _____

_____

_____

_____

OB LANKS

My first visit to the OB was on _____. Before settling on
DATE

Dr. _____, I spoke with _____ friends and _____
NAME   NUMBER   NUMBER

other doctor's offices. I chose Dr. _____ because
NAME

he/she is very _____ and _____. In the waiting
ADJECTIVE   ADJECTIVE

room I _____. During the appointment I complained
VERB

about _____. When the doctor informed me that
NOUN

while pregnant I should _____, but should not
NOUN

_____, I exclaimed "_____!" Before the
NOUN   EXPLETIVE

visit I felt _____. Now I feel _____ and so
ADJECTIVE   ADJECTIVE

_____. I'm glad that _____ came with me to
ADJECTIVE   NAME

the appointment.

I found out my due date! It is _____.
                                            DATE

DATE: / /

TIME: AM
PM

GLOW OR GAG:

BELLY: INCHES

CRANKOMETER:

half hormonal

wee bit
cranky

watch
out!

mellow
mommy

moody
maniac

GRIND AND THEN...
BUMP!

Knowing that my due date is _____, I believe the
date that the baby makin' happened was _____.

Where it happened: _____

Were you "trying"?

○ I've got an ovulation alarm set up on my smartphone.

○ I was just letting Mother Nature do her thing.

The situation was

○ Romantic and sexy.

○ Clinical and to the point.

○ Wild and spontaneous.

Could you tell it was a success?
Did you feel differently right away?

_____

_____

_____

_____

BUMP
IN THE ROAD

It was a bit trickier for me to get pregnant, so I took an alternate route.

○ In vitro

○ Artificial insemination

○ Other: _____

The procedure was

_____

_____

_____

_____

_____

_____

_____

_____

_____

_____

DATE: / /

TIME: AM
PM

GLOW OR GAG:

BELLY: INCHES

CRANKOMETER:

half hormonal

wee bit
cranky

watch
out!

mellow
mommy

moody
maniac

DATE: / /

TIME: AM
PM

BELLY: INCHES

GLOW OR GAG:

CRANKOMETER:

half hormonal

wee bit
cranky

watch
out!

mellow
mommy

moody
maniac

DATE: / /

TIME: ___ AM
        PM

GLOW or GAG:

BELLY: ___ INCHES

CRANKOMETER:

half hormonal

wee bit
cranky

watch
out!

mellow
mommy

moody
maniac

BUILD-A-BABY

IF YOU COULD SEND A REQUEST TO THE STORK, WHAT WOULD YOU ASK FOR?

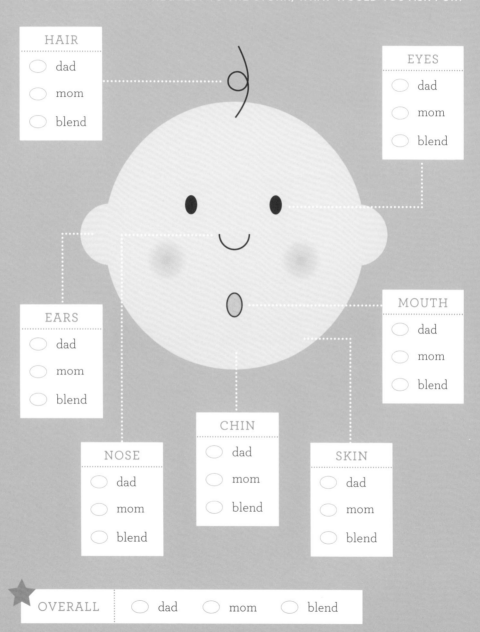

HAIR
- ○ dad
- ○ mom
- ○ blend

EYES
- ○ dad
- ○ mom
- ○ blend

EARS
- ○ dad
- ○ mom
- ○ blend

MOUTH
- ○ dad
- ○ mom
- ○ blend

NOSE
- ○ dad
- ○ mom
- ○ blend

CHIN
- ○ dad
- ○ mom
- ○ blend

SKIN
- ○ dad
- ○ mom
- ○ blend

OVERALL ○ dad ○ mom ○ blend

WHO'S YOUR
Daddy?

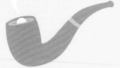

HAVE THE FATHER-TO-BE FILL IN THIS PAGE

I am your father, _____

But you can call me

Daddy   Dad   Dada   Pops   Mac Daddy   Other: _____

I make money to support you by being a _____

I hope you will grow up to be a _____

Some things I will teach you: _____

_____

_____

_____

_____

_____

_____

_____

Some things you will teach me: _____

_____

_____

_____

FRUITS

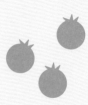

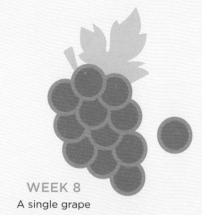

WEEK 7
A blueberry

WEEK 8
A single grape

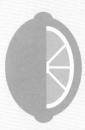

WEEK 11
A lime. Speaking of which,
wouldn't some key lime pie be
divine right about now?

WEEK 13
A peach. And your baby may
even be beginning to develop
fuzz on his/her head.

PACIFY YOUR WORRIES

It's normal to be nervous about the new life growing in your belly. You're not alone—interview an authority on the subject. Mom? Grandma? BFF?

Q _____
A _____
_____
_____

Q _____
A _____
_____
_____

Q _____
A _____
_____
_____

Q _____
A _____
_____
_____

DATE: / /

TIME: AM
PM

GLOW OR GAG:

BELLY: INCHES

CRANKOMETER:

half hormonal

wee bit
cranky

watch
out!

mellow
mommy

moody
maniac

PECULIAR
pregnancy dreams

Vivid dreams are just another "normal" part of this utterly unreal and exciting experience called pregnancy. They can be joyful and exhilarating, scandalous and sexy, totally frightening, or altogether odd. No matter what, you can rest assured that though they seem as real as can be, they're just your hormone-charged imagination running wild. Record one from this trimester here.

movie
NIGHT

FATHER OF THE BRIDE PART II

SHE'S HAVING A BABY

JUNIOR
(PREGNANT GUY ALERT!)

NINE MONTHS

WAITRESS

SHADE IN
THE MOVIES
YOU'VE SEEN

⟷

TWINS

BIG BUSINESS

PARENT TRAP
(HAYLEY MILLS CLASSIC)

THE PRESTIGE

THE MAN IN THE IRON MASK

double
FEATURE

DATE: / /

TIME: AM PM

GLOW OR GAG:

BELLY: INCHES

CRANKOMETER:

half hormonal

wee bit cranky

watch out!

mellow mommy

moody maniac

DATE: /   /

TIME: AM
                       PM

GLOW OR GAG:

BELLY: INCHES

CRANKOMETER:

half hormonal

wee bit
cranky   watch
                              out!

mellow   moody
mommy   maniac

CURRENT
cravings

Many women crave sour foods during pregnancy, while others go crazy for salty snacks. What foods do you currently find appetizing? Which ones repulse you? Make a list on the next page.

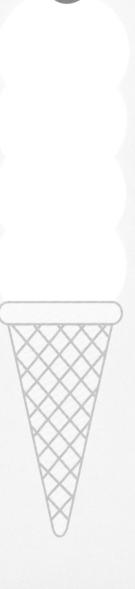

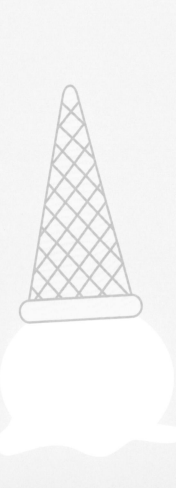

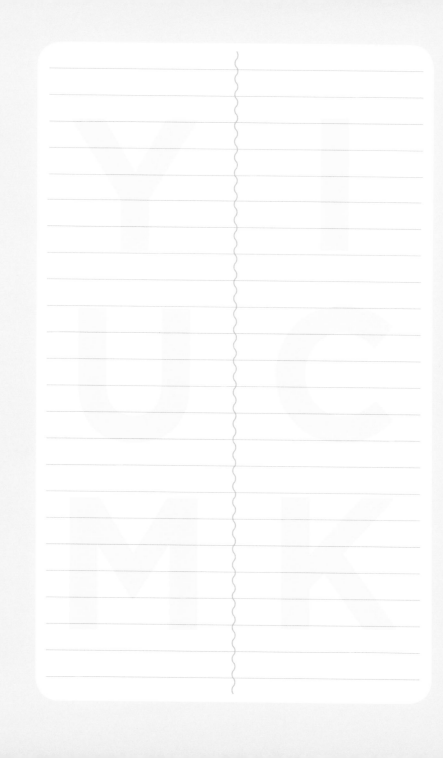

PREGNANCY:
bottle half empty...

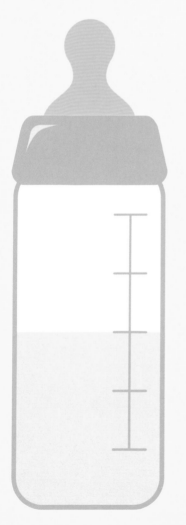

What I really miss that I
can't have right now...

My salami sandwich

Sushi

Glass of wine

Martini

Beer

Hot dogs

…or half full?

What I love about
being pregnant…

No period cramps!

Connecting with my baby

People hold the door for me

I have a better excuse to

indulge in treats

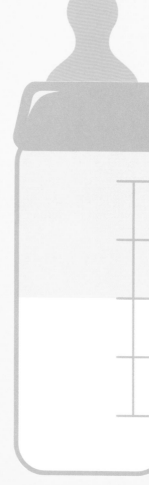

DATE: / /

TIME: AM
PM

GLOW OR GAG:

BELLY: INCHES

CRANKOMETER:

half hormonal

wee bit
cranky

watch
out!

mellow
mommy

moody
maniac

DATE: / /

TIME: _____ AM
PM

GLOW OR GAG:

BELLY: _____ INCHES

CRANKOMETER:

half hormonal

wee bit
cranky

watch
out!

mellow
mommy

moody
maniac

I'm not sure why, but I just have this feeling that it's...

- ☐ A girl.
- ☐ A boy.
- ☐ Both, in a set of fraternal twins.

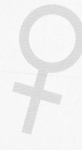

BATTLE OF THE
SEXES

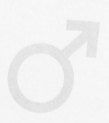

Will you find out the sex of your baby before the birth?

- ☐ Of course! I can't wait.
- ☐ No way! I love surprises.

Girl Names that Rock	What the Mean Kids Might Call Her

Boy Names that Rock	What the Mean Kids Might Call Him

TELL & SHOW

The rumor mill churns especially fast when it comes to baby news. Most couples like to control the when, who, and how of the big announcement. How did you go about the big reveal?

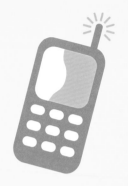

Date we told the grandparents-to-be.

Date we told any siblings-to-be.

Date that we started to share our great news with other relatives and friends. (Use chart at right for details.)

Date that I stopped dressing to hide the bump.

Date that I talked to my supervisor about maternity leave.

And lastly, when you're done spreading the news on a more personal basis...

Date that we went global and posted the news on Facebook/Twitter/a blog.

WHO	WHEN	💬	☎	✉

The most priceless reaction to the baby news was...

_____

_____

_____

_____

_____

Paste a copy of your first sonogram here.

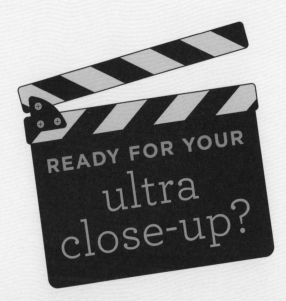

READY FOR YOUR
ultra
close-up?

DATE: / /

TIME: AM
PM

GLOW OR GAG:

BELLY: INCHES

CRANKOMETER:

half hormonal

wee bit
cranky

watch
out!

mellow
mommy

moody
maniac

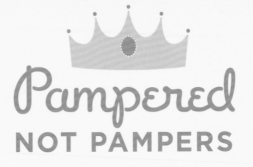

Pampered
NOT PAMPERS

Well, at least no diapers just yet. It's an unfortunate fact that you aren't going to feel like a beauty queen every day of your pregnancy, so you should at least treat yourself like one. A little me time can go a long way.

WHILE PREGGERS I WILL STILL MAINTAIN MY USUAL BEAUTY REGIMEN, WHICH INCLUDES:

Professional haircuts

Blow-outs

Manicures

Pedicures

Facials

Massages

Waxing

_____

_____

THINGS THAT I DON'T USUALLY PAY FOR, BUT WILL SPLURGE ON FOR NOW:

Professional haircuts

Blow-outs

Manicures

Pedicures

Facials

Massages

Waxing

_____

_____

I also get pampered at home by my husband, who is nice enough to: _____

_____

_____

HELLO

Second

TRIMESTER

FRUITS
OF YOUR LABOR 2

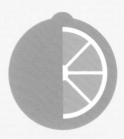

WEEK 16

A navel orange. How's your
navel doing? Is it protruding
more than before?

WEEK 19

Heirloom tomato

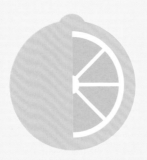

WEEK 21

A nice large grapefruit

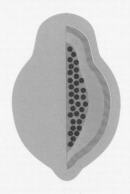

WEEK 25

About 19 weeks ago, your
baby was the size of a papaya
seed; now he/she's the size of
the whole fruit.

Pardon me
I'M PREGNANT

As your baby grows, controlling your bodily functions may become more difficult than you'd like. Other adults understand this and will be forgiving. Nonetheless, it can be totally embarrassing to let out a toot during a fancy dinner with your in-laws or the meeting about the big merger. Write about one such moment here. You want to forget it now, but you'll laugh about it later.

DATE: / /

TIME: AM
                PM

KICK COUNT:

not yet | once in a while | getting busy | totally footloose | future athlete

BELLY: INCHES

CRANKOMETER:

half hormonal

wee bit cranky   watch out!

mellow mommy   moody maniac

DATE: / /

TIME: AM
PM

KICK COUNT:

not yet | once in a while | getting busy | totally footloose | future athlete

BELLY: INCHES

CRANKOMETER:

half hormonal

wee bit cranky

watch out!

mellow mommy

moody maniac

DATE: / /

TIME: AM
          PM

KICK COUNT:

not yet   once in a while   getting busy   totally footloose   future athlete

BELLY: INCHES

CRANKOMETER:

half hormonal

wee bit cranky   watch out!

mellow mommy   moody maniac

PAPARAZZI

SCHEDULE A PHOTO SESSION WITH THE FATHER.
PASTE YOUR BEST SHOTS HERE.

FIRST FLUTTERS

The first time I felt my baby kick was _____

Did you think it was something else at first?

YES I was a little unsure. I thought maybe it was just gas.

NO It was unlike anything I'd ever felt.

NO This is not my first child, so I was familiar with the feeling.

How would you describe the sensation to a man?

_____

_____

_____

_____

_____

Baby is most active

When I'm trying to rest.

After I eat.

When I feel stressed out.

All the time.

DATE: / /

TIME: AM PM

KICK COUNT:

not yet | once in a while | getting busy | totally footloose | future athlete

BELLY: INCHES

CRANKOMETER:

half hormonal

wee bit cranky

watch out!

mellow mommy

moody maniac

DATE: / /

TIME: AM PM

KICK COUNT:

not yet | once in a while | getting busy | totally footloose | future athlete

BELLY: INCHES

CRANKOMETER:

half hormonal

wee bit cranky

watch out!

mellow mommy

moody maniac

PREGNANCY LOVES
company

Carrying a child is a shared experience for most women. You'll probably find that you have an instant connection with other pregnant ladies you "bump" into. Who are you bonding with over the little frustrations and big joys of pregnancy?

Friends who got pregnant around the same time as I did:

♥ _____

♥ _____

♥ _____

♥ _____

Friends I've met since becoming pregnant:

♥ _____

♥ _____

♥ _____

♥ _____

Celebrities or other prominent people who are currently pregnant:

♥ _____

♥ _____

♥ _____

DATE: / /

TIME: AM PM

KICK COUNT:

not yet   once in a while   getting busy   totally footloose   future athlete

BELLY: INCHES

CRANKOMETER:

half hormonal

wee bit cranky   watch out!

mellow mommy   moody maniac

DATE: / /

TIME: AM
       PM

KICK COUNT:

not yet | once in a while | getting busy | totally footloose | future athlete

BELLY: _____ INCHES

CRANKOMETER:

half hormonal

wee bit cranky   watch out!

mellow mommy   moody maniac

Paste a pic of yourself in your favorite
maternity outfit here.

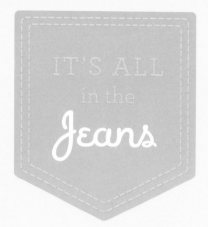

IT'S ALL
in the
Jeans

I realized it was time to shop for maternity clothes when

_____

_____

_____

_____

_____

_____

I purchased my first pair of maternity jeans on _____

The first day I had to wear them was _____

That made me feel _____

My favorite maternity brand/store is _____

I would describe my maternity style as:

○ Baby doll. I like A-line tops that don't touch my belly at all.

○ Bump-conscious. I wear things that hug the belly. I like my pregnant shape.

○ Easy-breezy. My preference is for flowy garments that graze the belly, but don't hug it.

My feet have swelled to a size _____, so . . .

○ I wear sneakers all the time. I'm a mom-to-be on the go.

○ I wear comfort-brand flats. Practical, but still feminine.

○ I rebought my favorite pumps in a larger size. Pregnant in heels describes me perfectly.

Have you been pouring over every pregnancy and child-rearing book around? Did you hit the bookstore or borrow it from a friend? Darken in the stars to rate what you've read.

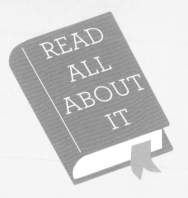

READ ALL ABOUT IT

TITLE	BUY?	BORROW?	RATE IT
			☆ ☆ ☆ ☆
			☆ ☆ ☆ ☆
			☆ ☆ ☆ ☆
			☆ ☆ ☆ ☆
			☆ ☆ ☆ ☆
			☆ ☆ ☆ ☆
			☆ ☆ ☆ ☆
			☆ ☆ ☆ ☆
			☆ ☆ ☆ ☆

DATE: / /

BELLY: _____ INCHES

TIME: _____ AM PM

KICK COUNT:

not yet | once in a while | getting busy | totally footloose | future athlete

CRANKOMETER:

wee bit cranky | half hormonal | watch out!

mellow mommy | moody maniac

DATE: / /

TIME: AM PM

KICK COUNT:

not yet · once in a while · getting busy · totally footloose · future athlete

BELLY: INCHES

CRANKOMETER:

half hormonal

wee bit cranky · watch out!

mellow mommy · moody maniac

Paste a copy of a second trimester sonogram here.

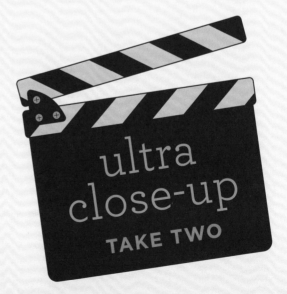

ultra
close-up

TAKE TWO

And the winner is...

- [ ] A girl (or girls).
- [ ] A boy (or boys).
- [ ] Both, in a set of multiples.
- [ ] No peeking. How suspenseful!

BATTLE OF THE
SEXES

Was your intuition on target?

- [ ] Of course.
- [ ] Not this time. This kid's a sneaky little guy/gal.

Names that are still in the running	What are the odds you'll pick it?

EVEN STRANGER
pregnancy dreams

Your morning sickness may have subsided after the first trimester, but the odd dreams are here to stay. Look for themes that change over time. Write about a dream experience from your second trimester here.

DATE: /   /

TIME: AM
                         PM

KICK COUNT:

not yet | once in a while | getting busy | totally footloose | future athlete

BELLY: INCHES

CRANKOMETER:

half hormonal

wee bit cranky   watch out!

mellow mommy   moody maniac

PRENATAL TEST

Have you read all the pregancy books that are out there cover to cover? Get out your #2 pencil and show off what you know. The answers are on the lower right, but no peeking!

The word *fetus* comes from the Latin meaning

- A tadpole
- B offspring
- C child

How long does it take for a fertilized egg to become a fetus?

- A 9 weeks after fertilization
- B it happens instantaneously
- C 20 weeks after fertilization

Can the human egg and/or sperm be seen by the naked eye?

- A both
- B the sperm, but not the egg
- C the egg, but not the sperm
- D neither

When do the family jewels form if it's a boy?

- A from the get-go
- B week 12
- C week 24
- D week 30

The last organ to fully develop is the

A heart

B kidneys

C lungs

You may become forgetful during pregnancy because

A you've got too much on your mind

B your brain temporarily shrinks

C what was the question?

It is normal for babies to do all of the following in utero EXCEPT

A pee

B suck his/her thumb

C poop

D hiccup

The hormone that helps you bond with your baby is called

A oxytocin

B adrenaline

C socuteareyou

ANSWERS: B, A, C, C, B, C, A

DATE: / /

TIME: AM PM

KICK COUNT:

not yet | once in a while | getting busy | totally footloose | future athlete

BELLY: INCHES

CRANKOMETER:

half hormonal

wee bit cranky | watch out!

mellow mommy | moody maniac

DATE: / /

BELLY: _____ INCHES

TIME: _____ AM
PM

CRANKOMETER:

KICK COUNT:

not yet | once in a while | getting busy | totally footloose | future athlete

half hormonal

wee bit cranky

watch out!

mellow mommy

moody maniac

CURRENT
cravings

How has your appetite changed since your first trimester? Have your cravings become stronger? How about stranger? What foods do you currently find irresistable? Which ones disgust you? Make a list on the next page.

DATE: / /

TIME: AM PM

KICK COUNT:

not yet | once in a while | getting busy | totally footloose | future athlete

BELLY: INCHES

CRANKOMETER:

half hormonal

wee bit cranky | watch out!

mellow mommy | moody maniac

BREAST
NEWS EVER?

So far, my breasts have gone from a

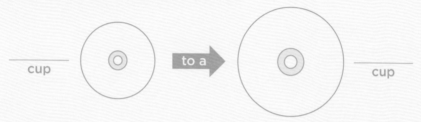

_____ cup **to a** cup

Did you buy new bras or are you letting your cups runneth over?

_____

_____

_____

_____

How about nursing bras? Have you checked those out yet?

_____

_____

How are you feeling about your expanding bustline?

◯ Thrilled! For once, I get to feel like a porn star.

◯ Less than excited. My boobs are sore and unwieldy.

◯ Doesn't make a difference to me either way, but my husband is over the moon about it.

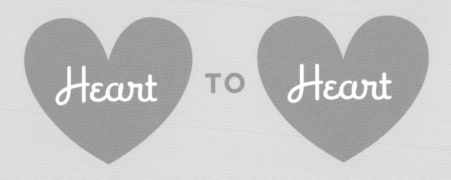

Heart TO Heart

Hearing my baby's heartbeat for the first time was

♥ Life-changing. It's finally sunk in that this thing is for real.

♥ Creepy. In a good way of course.

♥ Music to my ears. I wanted to listen all day.

How do you connect prenatally? Select all that apply.

♥ I play music for the bump.

♥ I speak to my unborn child so he/she will become familiar with my voice.

♥ I rest my hand on the bump and allow the dad to do the same.

♥ Other: _____

Have you ever felt your baby was reacting directly to something you said or did? Jot down your thoughts about that.

_____

_____

_____

_____

DATE: / /

TIME: ___ AM
PM

KICK COUNT:

not yet | once in a while | getting busy | totally footloose | future athlete

BELLY: ___ INCHES

CRANKOMETER:

half hormonal

wee bit cranky

watch out!

mellow mommy

moody maniac

DATE: / /

TIME: _____ AM
PM

KICK COUNT:

not yet • once in a while • getting busy • totally footloose • future athlete

BELLY: _____ INCHES

CRANKOMETER:

half hormonal

wee bit cranky   watch out!

mellow mommy   moody maniac

DATE: / /

TIME: AM PM

KICK COUNT:

not yet | once in a while | getting busy | totally footloose | future athlete

BELLY: INCHES

CRANKOMETER:

half hormonal

wee bit cranky

watch out!

mellow mommy

moody maniac

SO
SWEET!

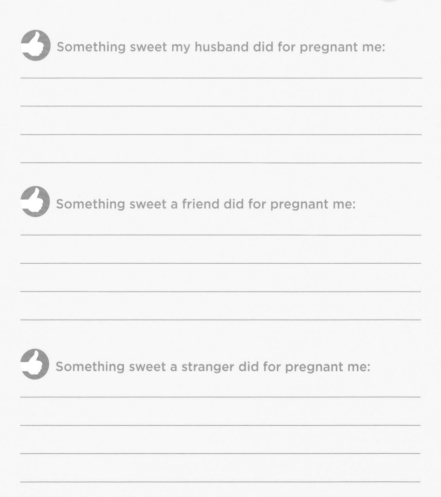

👍 Something sweet my husband did for pregnant me:

_____

_____

_____

_____

👍 Something sweet a friend did for pregnant me:

_____

_____

_____

_____

👍 Something sweet a stranger did for pregnant me:

_____

_____

_____

_____

HOW
RUDE!

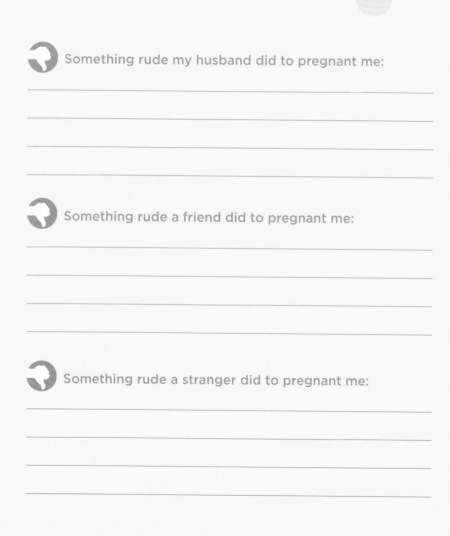

Something rude my husband did to pregnant me:

_____

_____

_____

_____

Something rude a friend did to pregnant me:

_____

_____

_____

_____

Something rude a stranger did to pregnant me:

_____

_____

_____

_____

DATE: / /

TIME: AM PM

BELLY: INCHES

KICK COUNT:

not yet | once in a while | getting busy | totally footloose | future athlete

CRANKOMETER:

half hormonal

wee bit cranky

watch out!

mellow mommy

moody maniac

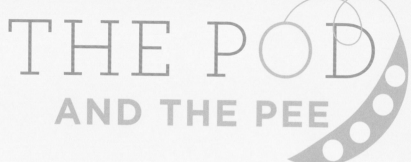

THE POD
AND THE PEE

As baby gets bigger he/she will start to crowd your bladder.
Have you had any embarassing accidents or near accidents as
a result of lessened bladder control?

_____

_____

_____

_____

_____

Have you been doing your kegels?

- Can I not and say I did?
- Every chance I get. Want to keep things nice and tight.
- I'm doing them right now. Wink, wink.

**What about other less private physical activities to keep you
in shape for the big event? Pregnancy yoga? Water aerobics?**

_____

_____

_____

_____

THE
babymooners

Many mommies-to-be find time during the second trimester to take a vacay. The itsy-bitsy teeny-weeny yellow polka-dot bikini may no longer be an option, but don't let that stop you from getting some quality rest and relaxation. Where did you go? Who was your travel companion? Use this space to write about the fantastic time you had.

_____

_____

_____

_____

_____

_____

_____

_____

_____

_____

_____

_____

DATE: / /

TIME: AM PM

KICK COUNT:

not yet | once in a while | getting busy | totally footloose | future athlete

BELLY: INCHES

CRANKOMETER:

half hormonal
wee bit cranky
watch out!
mellow mommy
moody maniac

CRYBABY

As you know by now, being pregnant can send you on an emotional roller coaster. Have you noticed yourself tearing up during commercials you'd normally find silly? Record some situations or circumstances that you were surprised sent you into a sob-fest.

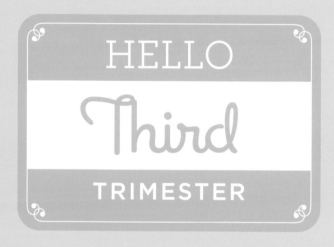

HELLO

Third

TRIMESTER

FRUITS

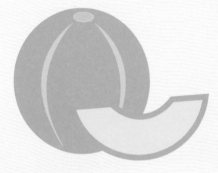

WEEK 33

A honeydew. Do you have a "honey-do" list prepared so your honey knows how he can help?

WEEK 30

A pineapple, but not so prickly

WEEK 37 AND BEYOND

A watermelon—YIKES! Just like Jennifer Grey in *Dirty Dancing*, you can now say, "I carried a watermelon."

DATE: / /

TIME: AM / PM

BELLY: INCHES

KICK COUNTDOWN:

up all night — still movin' — chilling out — a little legroom — outgrown my home

CRANKOMETER:

half hormonal

wee bit cranky — watch out!

mellow mommy — moody maniac

PREP YOUR
CRIB

For most mommies, the nesting impulse hits sometime during the second trimester and continues through the third. This is Mother Nature's way of getting you to prepare a proper living space for baby. This can include urges to baby-proof, clean, and decorate. How are you sprucing up your nest?

TO DO

- ☐ _____
- ☐ _____
- ☐ _____
- ☐ _____
- ☐ _____
- ☐ _____
- ☐ _____
- ☐ _____
- ☐ _____
- ☐ _____
- ☐ _____
- ☐ _____
- ☐ _____

TO BUY

- ☐ _____
- ☐ _____
- ☐ _____
- ☐ _____
- ☐ _____

TO BORROW

- ☐ _____
- ☐ _____
- ☐ _____
- ☐ _____
- ☐ _____

Before

Paste a "before" picture of baby's space here.

Paste an "after" picture of baby's space here.

After

DATE: / /

TIME: _____ AM
PM

KICK COUNTDOWN:

up all night · still movin' · chilling out · a little legroom · outgrown my home

BELLY: _____ INCHES

CRANKOMETER:

half hormonal

wee bit cranky   watch out!

mellow mommy   moody maniac

DATE: / /

TIME: ___ AM PM

KICK COUNTDOWN:

up all night · still movin' · chilling out · a little legroom · outgrown my home

BELLY: ___ INCHES

ZZZZMETER:

baby's bugging me — restless — well rested — not a wink — sleeping beauty

_____
_____
_____
_____
_____
_____
_____
_____
_____
_____
_____
_____
_____
_____
_____
_____
_____
_____
_____
_____
_____
_____
_____
_____
_____

BREATHE easier

MY FIRST BIRTHING CLASS

Date: /   /   Location: Instructor: .

Topics covered by the instructor:

_____

_____

_____

_____

_____

My impressions of what we learned:

_____

_____

_____

_____

_____

MAKING THE GRADE

I deserve an   (A)   (B)   (C)

Why?

_____

_____

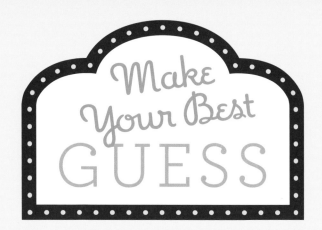

Make Your Best GUESS

PREDICT...	YOUR GUESS	THE DAD'S GUESS
baby's weight		
baby's length		
baby's birth date		
time of birth		
duration of labor		
if baby will have hair or not		
if you cry upon seeing your child		
if baby's daddy will cry upon seeing his child		
the baby's gender (if still unknown)		

Paste a copy of a third trimester or final sonogram here.

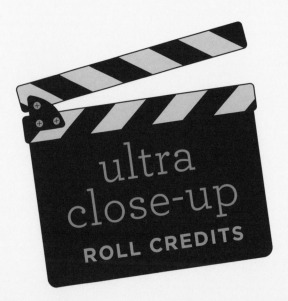

ultra
close-up
ROLL CREDITS

DATE: / /

TIME: AM PM

BELLY: INCHES

KICK COUNTDOWN:

up all night

still movin'

chilling out

a little legroom

outgrown my home

ZZZZMETER:

restless

baby's bugging me

well rested

not a wink

sleeping beauty

DATE: /   /

TIME: AM
               PM

BELLY: _____ INCHES

KICK COUNTDOWN:

up all night — still movin' — chilling out — a little legroom — outgrown my home

CRANKOMETER:

half hormonal

wee bit cranky   watch out!

mellow mommy   moody maniac

DATE: / /

TIME: AM PM

BELLY: INCHES

KICK COUNTDOWN:

up all night
still movin'
chilling out
a little legroom
outgrown my home

ZZZZMETER:

baby's bugging me
restless
well rested
not a wink
sleeping beauty

SHOWERED
with gifts

NAME OF HOST:

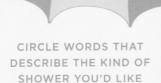

CIRCLE WORDS THAT DESCRIBE THE KIND OF SHOWER YOU'D LIKE

Modern

Mega-Girly

Tea Party

Co-ed

Gourmet

Comfort Food

Silly Games

Cute

Brunch

Diaper Cake

Spa Day

Intimate

Rowdy

Mocktails

Sophisticated

Girl Talk

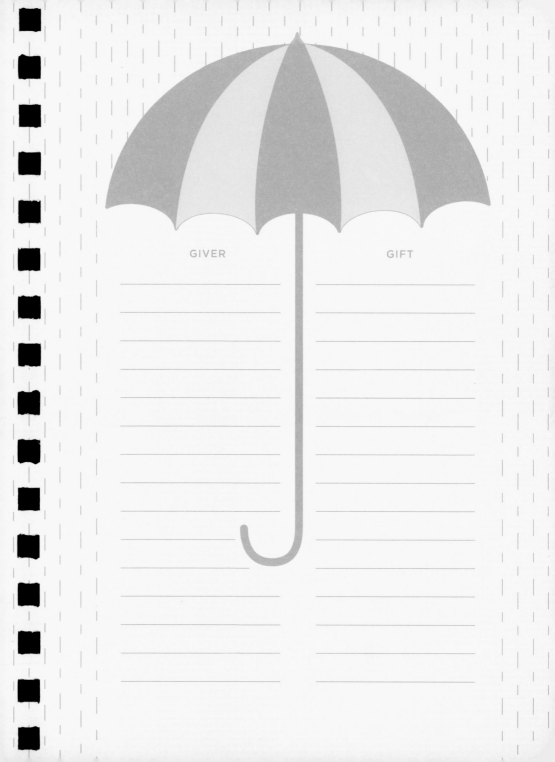

GIVER

GIFT

KICK COUNTDOWN:

up all night — still movin' — chilling out — a little legroom — outgrown my home

half hormonal

wee bit cranky   watch out!

mellow mommy   moody maniac

DATE: / /

TIME: AM PM

BELLY: INCHES

ZZZZMETER:

KICK COUNTDOWN:

up all night

still movin'

chilling out

a little legroom

outgrown my home

restless

baby's bugging me

well rested

not a wink

sleeping beauty

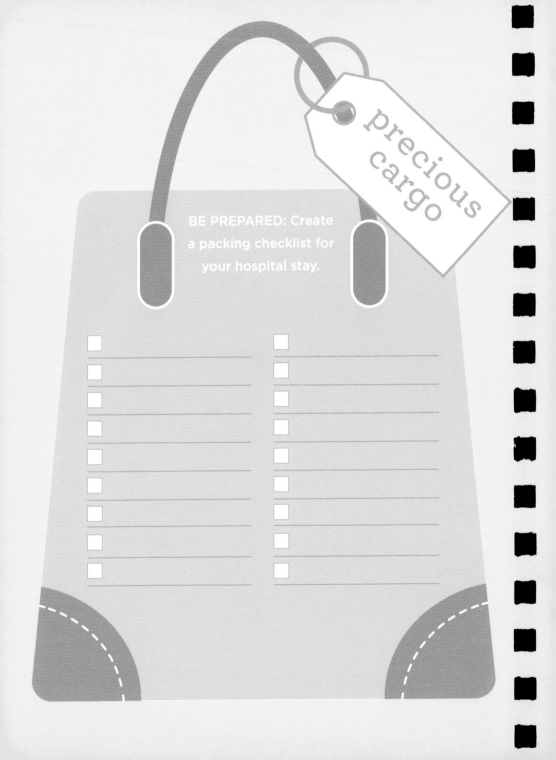

BE PREPARED: Create a packing checklist for your hospital stay.

precious cargo

DATE: / /

TIME: AM
       PM

KICK COUNTDOWN:

up all night | still movin' | chilling out | a little legroom | outgrown my home

BELLY: INCHES

ZZZZMETER:

                    restless

baby's   well
bugging   rested
me

not a   sleeping
wink   beauty

DELIVERY ROUTE

Even if you're not the planning type, it is a good idea to put some thought into your delivery. Unless you're being induced, labor can start anywhere, anytime. Ready or not, here comes baby!

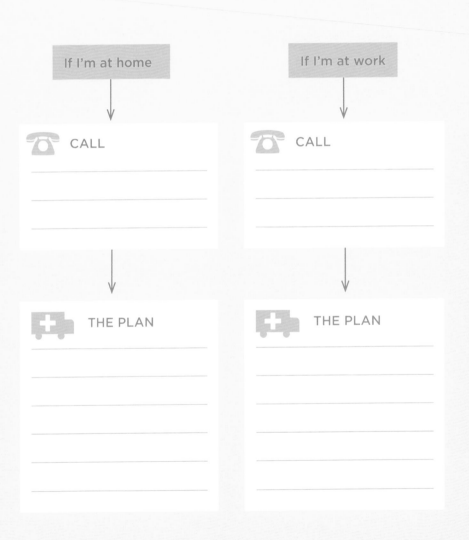

If I'm at home

☎ CALL

_____
_____
_____

🚑 THE PLAN

_____
_____
_____
_____
_____

If I'm at work

☎ CALL

_____
_____
_____

🚑 THE PLAN

_____
_____
_____
_____
_____

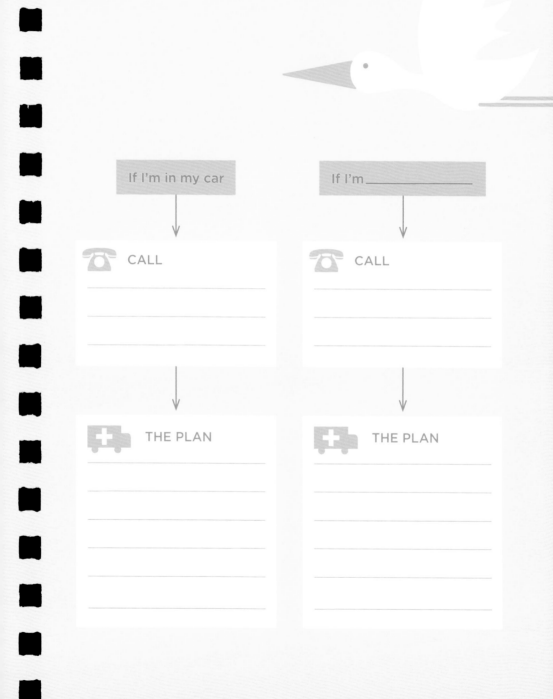

If I'm in my car

If I'm_____

☎ CALL

☎ CALL

🚑 THE PLAN

🚑 THE PLAN

DATE: / /

TIME: AM PM

KICK COUNTDOWN:

up all night · still movin' · chilling out · a little legroom · outgrown my home

BELLY: _____ INCHES

CRANKOMETER:

half hormonal

wee bit cranky

watch out!

mellow mommy

moody maniac

DATE: / /

TIME: ___ AM
PM

KICK COUNTDOWN:

up all night

still movin'

chilling out

a little legroom

outgrown my home

BELLY: _____ INCHES

ZZZZMETER:

restless

baby's bugging me

well rested

not a wink

sleeping beauty

BUN'S
ALMOST DONE

Paste a few bump photos from mid to
late third trimester on these pages.
Don't forget to jot down the date next
to each picture.

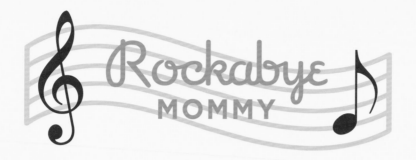

Rockabye MOMMY

You've probably noticed it has become more and more difficult to sleep as your pregnancy progresses. Not surprising given your ever-changing bump. What do you do to lull yourself to sleep?

Are you using a preganancy pillow?

YES I love it, but my husband feels a little replaced by it.

NO It came highly recommended, but it didn't do it for me.

What bugs you the most at night?

I have to pee every hour. Annoying!

I used to sleep on my stomach and I miss that.

Mostly stress, I think. Surprisingly, I'm not too uncomfortable physically.

I'm having odd nightmares that come out of nowhere about my husband cheating on me with species from outer space.

What recommendations have you gotten from doctors and friends about getting to sleep more easily?

_____

_____

_____

What have you discovered that most helps you catch your ZZZs?

_____

_____

_____

_____

_____

_____

midnight
SHOWING

Can't sleep? Watch one of these movies about
parenting. Do yourself a favor and pick a
comedy. Now's not the time to take on *Sophie's
Choice* if you ever want to get to sleep.

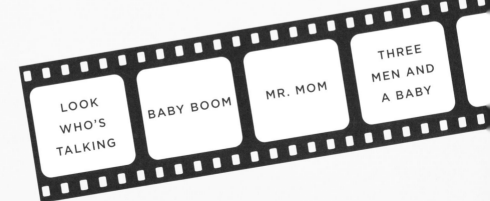

LOOK WHO'S TALKING

BABY BOOM

MR. MOM

THREE MEN AND A BABY

DATE: / /

TIME: AM PM

KICK COUNTDOWN:

up all night | still movin' | chilling out | a little legroom | outgrown my home

BELLY: INCHES

CRANKOMETER:

half hormonal

wee bit cranky

watch out!

mellow mommy

moody maniac

DATE: / /

TIME: AM
PM

KICK COUNTDOWN:

up all night · still movin' · chilling out · a little legroom · outgrown my home

BELLY: INCHES

ZZZZMETER:

restless

baby's bugging me · well rested

not a wink · sleeping beauty

Father

KNOWS BEST

Have the dad-to-be jot down some fatherly advice below.

_____

_____

_____

_____

_____

_____

_____

_____

_____

_____

_____

_____

_____

_____

_____

_____

_____

K N O W S   Mother   B E S T

Jot down some of your motherly advice here.

_____

_____

_____

_____

_____

_____

_____

_____

_____

_____

_____

_____

_____

DATE: / /

TIME: AM
PM

KICK COUNTDOWN:

up all night

still movin'

chilling out

a little legroom

outgrown my home

BELLY: INCHES

CRANKOMETER:

half hormonal

wee bit cranky

watch out!

mellow mommy

moody maniac

DATE: / /

TIME: AM PM

KICK COUNTDOWN:

up all night · still movin' · chilling out · a little legroom · outgrown my home

BELLY: _____ INCHES

ZZZZMETER:

restless

baby's bugging me

well rested

not a wink

sleeping beauty

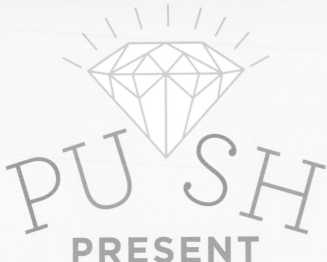

PUSH
PRESENT

Do you want one?

YES I'm giving my husband the gift of a child. The least he could do is give me some jewelry to commemorate our new baby and my 9-plus months of hard work.

NO I'm already getting a priceless gift. I don't need anything else. Some flowers would be nice, though.

If you said yes, make a wish list.

⭐ _____   ⭐ _____

⭐ _____   ⭐ _____

⭐ _____   ⭐ _____

If you said no, is there something else you had in mind for the money your husband had set aside for the push present?

⭐ _____

_____

DATE: / /

TIME: AM
                          PM

BELLY: INCHES

ZZZZMETER:

KICK COUNTDOWN:

up all night · still movin' · chilling out · a little legroom · outgrown my home

restless

baby's bugging me · well rested

not a wink · sleeping beauty

DATE: /   /

TIME: AM
                         PM

KICK COUNTDOWN:

up all night · still movin' · chilling out · a little legroom · outgrown my home

BELLY: INCHES

CRANKOMETER:

half hormonal

wee bit cranky   watch out!

mellow mommy   moody maniac

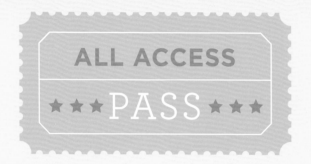

ALL ACCESS

★ ★ ★ PASS ★ ★ ★

These lucky people get to witness the miracle I will perform:

★ _____   ★ _____

★ _____   ★ _____

★ _____   ★ _____

Is videotaping the performance allowed?

YES I want to be able to watch an instant replay.

NO I'll capture this memory with a mental picture, not a moving one.

What about flash photography?

⬭ Snap away the whole time. I'll edit out what I don't like.

⬭ Only after the baby is born and I've had a chance to brush my hair.

⬭ If I so much as see a camera, I'll_____.

Would you like music to set the mood?

⬭ A melodic and soothing playlist that I've put on my iPod.

⬭ An inspirational soundtrack that includes the themes from
Chariots of Fire and _Rocky_.

⬭ No way. Though there might be screaming, this is _not_ a concert.

⬭ Other. I'd like to hear_____.

DATE: / /

TIME: AM
PM

KICK COUNTDOWN:

up all night | still movin' | chilling out | a little legroom | outgrown my home

BELLY: INCHES

CRANKOMETER:

half hormonal

wee bit cranky

watch out!

mellow mommy

moody maniac

READY TO
POP

Take one last picture before your due date and paste it here. Soon you'll be able to start the deflating process.

DATE: / /

TIME: AM PM

KICK COUNTDOWN:

up all night · still movin' · chilling out · a little legroom · outgrown my home

BELLY: INCHES

ZZZZMETER:

restless

baby's bugging me · well rested

not a wink · sleeping beauty

DATE: / /

BELLY: _____ INCHES

TIME: _____ AM PM

KICK COUNTDOWN:

up all night | still movin' | chilling out | a little legroom | outgrown my home

ZZZZMETER:

restless

baby's bugging me

well rested

not a wink

sleeping beauty

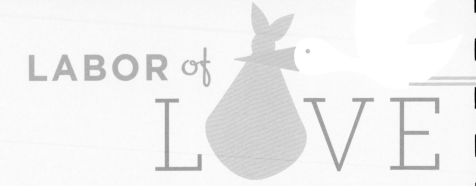

LABOR of LOVE

Hospital or home birth? _____

Doctor, doula, and/or midwife? _____

Epidural? Why or why not? _____

_____

/	:	} Date and time of your first official contraction.
/	:	} Date and time when your water broke.
/	:	} Date and time when you arrived at the hospital.
/	:	} Date you were induced or had your scheduled C-section.

Tell your birth story here. (Warning: If you write about how labor was a piece of cake, other women *will* be jealous.)

_____

_____

_____

_____

_____

_____

_____

_____

_____

_____

_____

_____

_____

_____

_____

_____

_____

_____

_____

_____

Paste a picture from the delivery experience
here. It could be taken before delivery, during,
or after. It's your call. It might not be your
birthday, but it's *the* birth day, so it's your day.

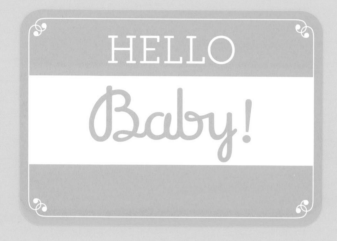

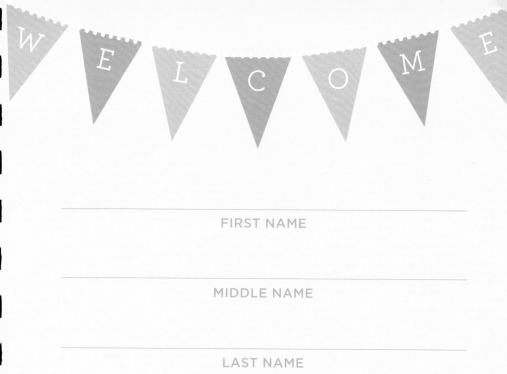

FIRST NAME

MIDDLE NAME

LAST NAME

DATE

TIME

POUNDS, OUNCES

INCHES

BIRTHPLACE

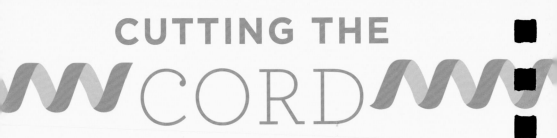

CUTTING THE CORD

The person who did the honors was _____

How did he or she handle it?

- Like a pro. I knew I was in good hands.
- Like a wuss. Bring on the smelling salts.
- Like a maniac. The way he/she wielded the clamp/scissors reminded me of a horror movie.

Cutting the umbilical cord separates your baby from you physically, but it signifies an emotional change, too. Write down your feelings about having your baby in the world with you, instead of in your belly.

_____

_____

_____

_____

_____

_____

_____

_____

DATE: / /

MOM MOOD:

TIME: AM PM

MILKMETER:

MINI MOOD MONITOR:

all smiles   content   grouchy

half tank

replenishing
supply

full jugs

empty

time to
pump

DATE: / /

TIME: AM
PM

MOM MOOD:

MILKMETER:

MINI MOOD MONITOR:

all smiles   content   grouchy

half tank

replenishing
supply

full jugs

empty

time to
pump

DATE: / /

MOM MOOD:

TIME: AM PM

MILKMETER:

MINI MOOD MONITOR:

all smiles   content   grouchy

half tank

replenishing
supply

full jugs

empty

time to
pump

FIRST IMPRESSIONS

DECIDE WHO BABY RESEMBLES MOST PHYSICALLY.

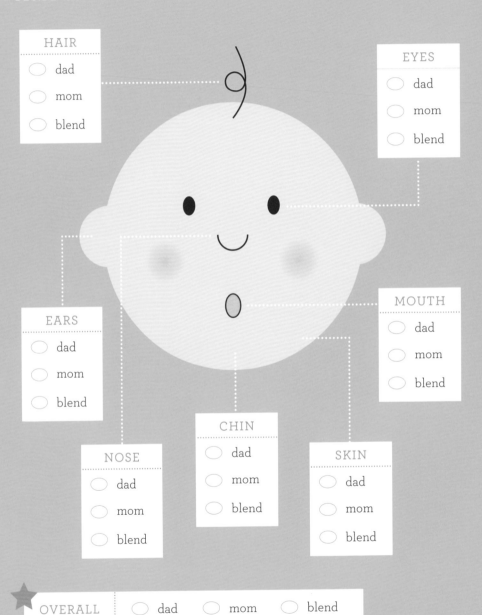

HAIR
- ○ dad
- ○ mom
- ○ blend

EYES
- ○ dad
- ○ mom
- ○ blend

EARS
- ○ dad
- ○ mom
- ○ blend

MOUTH
- ○ dad
- ○ mom
- ○ blend

NOSE
- ○ dad
- ○ mom
- ○ blend

CHIN
- ○ dad
- ○ mom
- ○ blend

SKIN
- ○ dad
- ○ mom
- ○ blend

OVERALL   ○ dad   ○ mom   ○ blend

WHAT DOES HIS/HER TEMPERAMENT REVEAL ABOUT HIS/HER
PERSONALITY? RECORD YOUR IMPRESSIONS ON THESE SLIDING
SCALES. LOOK BACK AT THIS PAGE IN A FEW MONTHS AND SEE
IF YOUR ASSESSMENT IS STILL ON TARGET.

FUSSY ···········|············|············|············|············ HAPPY-GO-LUCKY

HIGH ENERGY ···········|············|············|············|············ SLEEPY HEAD

NEEDY ···········|············|············|············|············ INDEPENDENT

CONSTANT CRYING ···········|············|············|············|············ SURPRISINGLY FEW TEARS

OVERALL PERSONALITY WILL BE MORE LIKE

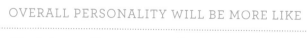

◯ dad   ◯ mom   ◯ too soon to say

Splish Splash

BABY'S FIRST BATH

Paste a picture of this special bonding experience here. Write a cute caption in the space below.

_____

_____

FILLING
STATION

Breast, bottle, or a bit of both? _____

Explain your choice: _____
_____
_____
_____
_____

What's your impression of pumping?
CIRCLE ALL THAT APPLY

awkward   OUCH!

strange, but fine   total time-suck

multitasking opportunity

Have you sprung a leak? _____
_____
_____
_____

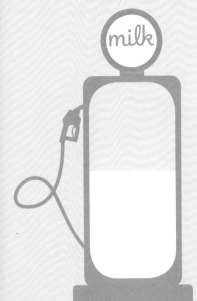
milk

MILK 'EM

FOR ALL THEY'RE WORTH

How do you feel about your extra-inflated assets? Talk about some wanted or unwanted attention you've gotten with them.

_____

_____

_____

_____

_____

_____

_____

_____

_____

_____

_____

_____

_____

_____

DIAPER
genie

Use this page to record who makes the most dirty diapers magically disappear over the course of a few days. Draw stars on the diapers to keep a tally. Reward the person with the most stars. Especially if it's you!

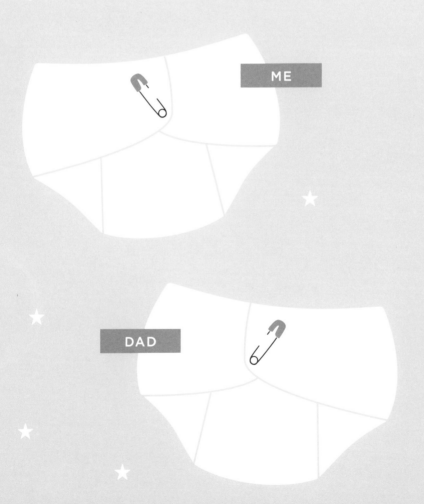

ME

DAD

GRANDPARENT

OLDER BRO
OR SIS

THE
BOOGEYMAN

DATE: / /

MOM MOOD:

TIME: AM
            PM

MILKMETER:

MINI MOOD MONITOR:

all smiles   content   grouchy

half tank

replenishing
supply

full jugs

empty

time to
pump

DATE: /   /

MOM MOOD:

TIME: AM
                        PM

MILKMETER:

MINI MOOD MONITOR:

all smiles   content   grouchy

half tank

replenishing
supply

full jugs

empty

time to
pump

DATE: / /

MOM MOOD:

TIME: AM PM

MILKMETER:

MINI MOOD MONITOR:

all smiles   content   grouchy

half tank

replenishing supply

full jugs

empty

time to pump

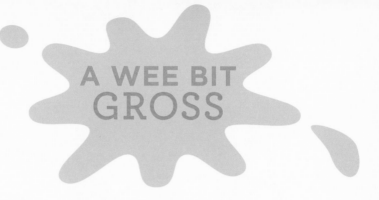

A WEE BIT GROSS

Let's face it. Babies are messy. Luckily for us, Mother Nature had her thinking cap on: Babies are so cute that you won't mind cleaning up after them. Even their poo is just darling. Okay… maybe it's not *that* great, but it's bearable. Write a pee, poo, cord-stump, or spit-up story here.

DATE: / /

MOM MOOD:

TIME: _____ AM
              PM

MINI MOOD MONITOR:

all smiles   content   grouchy

MILKMETER:

half tank

replenishing
supply   full jugs

empty   time to
                          pump

DATE: /   /

MOM MOOD:

TIME: AM
                        PM

MILKMETER:

MINI MOOD MONITOR:

all smiles   content   grouchy

half tank

replenishing
supply

full jugs

empty

time to
pump

I LOVE YOU THIS
MUCH

Attempt the impossible. Try to put your ever-expanding
love for your new baby into words.

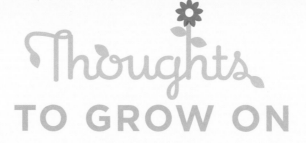

Thoughts
TO GROW ON

I can't believe how fast he/she has grown! _____
NAME OF BABY

is now _____ weeks and _____ days old. He/She
NUMBER   NUMBER

weighs _____ pounds and is _____ inches long.
NUMBER   NUMBER

He/She is very _____ and _____ .
ADJECTIVE   ADJECTIVE

I like it when we _____ together.
DESCRIPTION OF ACTIVITY

My friends and family think he/she is the _____
SUPERLATIVE

baby they've ever seen.

That whole "they grow up so fast" saying has truth to it. Make
a list of some of the things you look forward to experiencing
with your child as he/she grows up.

_____

_____

_____

_____

_____

_____

_____

If you thought pregnancy was a wild and amazing experience … get ready for parenting!

Published in 2013 by Stewart, Tabori & Chang
An imprint of ABRAMS

Copyright © 2013 Alissa Faden

Library of Congress Control Number: 2011935055
ISBN: 978-1-58479-965-8

Editor: Wesley Royce
Designer: Alissa Faden
Production Managers: Anet Sirna-Bruder and Tina Cameron

The text of this book was composed in Archer, Gotham, and Apricot.

Printed and bound in China

10 9 8 7 6 5 4 3

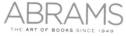

THE ART OF BOOKS SINCE 1949

115 West 18th Street
New York, NY 10011
www.abramsbooks.com